Wellness Made Easy

101 TIPS FOR BETTER HEALTH

from the

University of California, Berkeley Wellness Letter

This book is based on material published in the *University of California, Berkeley Wellness Letter* in association with the School of Public Health, University of California at Berkeley.

Printed in the U.S.A. 10 9 8 7 6 5 4 3

CONTENTS

INTRODUCTION

The idea of "good health" is changing. That's why the editors have chosen the word "wellness" for this book and for the *University of California, Berkeley Wellness Letter.*

Wellness isn't simply the absence of sickness, and health care isn't simply an effort to cure disease. Wellness is a way of living that emphasizes such preventive measures as eating a healthful diet, making regular exercise an enjoyable part of your life, and cultivating self-awareness. It means having the will to take charge of your own health.

Wellness does not mean "alternative" medicine (fad diets, herbal medications, or similar measures). Nor is it a substitute for medical care. Wellness does mean reducing your risk for chronic disease, preventing and treating injuries, banishing environmental and safety hazards from your home and workplace, and eliminating unnecessary trips to the doctor—but making the best use of the health-care system when you need it.

The information in the following pages will set you on the road to wellness. All of it is taken from the *Wellness Letter* and is backed by the consensus of the researchers and clinicians at the School of Public Health at the University of California at Berkeley, one of the nation's leading research and teaching institutions in this field. Their recommendations have emerged from reviews of thousands of scientific studies. Their intent is to supply guidelines that are clear, practical and up to date.

The premise of wellness is that you can live a long, healthy, and active life. All you need is the desire to do so—and the right information on which to base your actions.

Nutrition

EATING FOR HEALTH AND LONGEVITY

1 Buy cheap: Highly nutritious foods rich in vitamins, minerals, and fiber are often low in cost. Among these foods are potatoes, bananas, carrots, rice, whole-wheat flour, and dried beans—the sort of high-fiber, low-fat foods that nutritionists now recommend. Such unprocessed foods also tend to come with minimal packaging—an environmental plus.

2 Clean up your recipes. Sticking to a healthy diet is a matter of creative cooking. Many standard recipes call for more sugar, salt, or fat than is necessary:

- Try using half the amount of sugar called for.
- Substitute skim milk (evaporated skim milk is as thick as cream), low-fat or nonfat yogurt, or low-fat cottage cheese (puréed in a blender with a little lemon juice) for whole milk, cream, or sour cream.
- Use two egg whites instead of a whole egg.
- Use herbs and lemon or lime juice for seasoning vegetables in place of butter.
- Use nonstick pans.
- Marinate meat, poultry, and fish in herb-flavored vinegar, wine, lemon juice, well-seasoned broth, or low-sodium soy sauce instead of oil-based marinades.

3 Steer clear of fad diets. Quick weight-loss plans don't work. The weight you lose at the start is almost inevitably water, not fat. Moreover, most of these diets don't offer realistic lifetime eating plans. Permanent changes in eating habits and regular aerobic exercise are the keys to weight loss. Pass up any diet plan that:

- Guarantees you'll lose a certain number of pounds a week—especially more than two pounds.
- Emphasizes a particular food above all others.
- Recommends vitamin or mineral supplements to compensate for nutrients missing in the diet (be especially wary if supplements are sold along with the diet plan).
- Omits one food group or major nutrient, such as carbohydrates.
- Uses fanciful theories to explain how a combination of certain foods can improve your health and lead to weight loss.
- Recommends a total daily intake of less than 1,200 calories, unless you're under medical supervision.

4 Beware of unhealthy "health" foods. Many unhealthy foods have a healthy ring to them, but are actually loaded with fat, cholesterol, and/or calories. For example, although all muffins made with bran contain some fiber, they may not be good fiber sources. Most bakery or deli muffins have far more hydrogenated oil, sugar, and eggs than they do oat or wheat bran. If the muffin weighs heavily in your hand and has a sticky surface, it is likely to have as many calories and as much fat as any cupcake or doughnut. This is also true of carrot cakes and banana breads. While carrots and bananas are healthful foods, the baked goods that bear their names are almost inevitably dense and moist, usually signs of a high fat content.

5 Spare yourself the expense of vitamin and mineral supplements. People rarely need nutritional supplements; most people can easily get all the vitamins and minerals they need from a well-rounded diet. If the American diet were seriously deficient in nutrients, deficiency diseases such as beriberi and scurvy would be rampant. Besides, vitamin and mineral supplements cannot replace food or turn a junk-food diet into a healthy one. In fact, supplementation can be dangerous: megadoses of certain vitamins and minerals are potentially toxic. Certain categories of people, however, are more likely to suffer from vitamin deficiencies. You should seek nutritional advice if you smoke, are pregnant, are 65 or over, take aspirin frequently, or have more than two alcoholic drinks a day.

6 **Be a semi-vegetarian.** A semi-vegetarian is someone who supplements a steady diet of vegetables, grains, legumes, fruit, and dairy products with occasional moderate servings of beef, poultry, and fish. The potential health benefits of a semi-vegetarian diet are many: a lowered risk for heart disease, cancer, and diabetes, lower blood cholesterol and blood pressure levels, the maintenance of a proper weight, and fewer digestive complaints such as constipation. Most low-fat, "heart-healthy" meal plans are essentially semi-vegetarian diets, as are many ethnic cuisines.

7 **Check food labels for hidden sources of sodium.** When most people think about cutting back on sodium they think about cutting back on salt, but salt and sodium are not interchangeable terms. Sodium, in various guises, is routinely added to packaged foods. If you're trying to reduce the amount of sodium in your diet, be on the lookout for the following when reading labels: baking powder, baking soda, soy sauce, brine, garlic salt, onion salt, kelp, monosodium glutamate (MSG), sea salt, sodium chloride (table salt), sodium citrate, sodium nitrate, sodium phosphate, and sodium saccharin.

8 Microwave to retain nutrients. In conventional cooking, heat is applied from the outside and gradually penetrates food, but microwaves cook the interior of foods directly by causing water molecules to vibrate, thus creating heat. Because microwaves act on the water content, microwaving is a kind of steaming—an excellent way to preserve nutrients. Some studies have shown that microwaving conserves more B vitamins (such as thiamin and riboflavin) and vitamin C than conventional cooking methods.

9 Cut back on fat. Fat should contribute no more than 30 percent of your total daily calories. This doesn't mean that every food you eat must derive less than 30 percent of its calories from fat, but that you should balance higher-fat foods with plenty of low-fat foods so that your *total* intake of fat accounts for no more than 30 percent of the calories you eat on a given day. To reduce the amount of fat you eat:

- Substitute grains or legumes for meat in some meals.
- Select lean meats and eat smaller portions of them (three to five ounces).
- Trim all visible fat from meat and remove the skin from poultry before cooking.
- Choose low-fat or nonfat dairy products.
- Limit your intake of fats and oils by cutting down on butter, cream, lard, salad dressings, and foods made with coconut, palm, or palm kernel oil, or hydrogenated vegetable oil.
- Use nonstick cooking spray instead of butter or oil whenever possible.
- Broil, bake, boil, or microwave foods instead of frying them.
- Moderate your use of fat-laden snack foods, such as potato chips, corn chips, cookies, cakes, and pastries.

10 Calculate your percentage of fat calories. To determine the percentage of calories derived from fat in a particular food, you need to know the number of calories and grams of fat in a serving. This information is printed on most food labels. Multiply the grams of fat in a serving by 9 (there are 9 calories in a gram of fat). Then divide that number by the total calories in the serving. The formula is (grams of fat x 9) ÷ (total calories). For example: a tablespoon of peanut butter has 8 grams of fat and 95 calories. So 8 x 9 = 72, divided by the number of calories (95) equals 0.76, or 76 percent calories from fat. An easy way to roughly evaluate the fat content of a food is to multiply the grams of fat by 9; if the result is more than a third of the total calories, the food is relatively high in fat.

11 Eat low-fat to keep your weight in check. Some studies have suggested that it's not just the number of calories you eat that causes weight gain or loss, but also what type of foods those calories come from. Excess weight seems to be linked to fat consumption, independent of calorie intake. Researchers have found evidence that the body may be able to convert dietary fat into body fat with greater ease than it can convert carbohydrates into body fat. One study suggests that if you consume 100 excess *carbohydrate* calories, 23 of the calories will be used simply to process the food, and thus only 77 of them will end up being stored as body fat. But when you eat 100 excess *fat* calories, your body uses only three of the calories to process the food, and so 97 calories end up being stored as body fat.

12 Take steps to prevent food poisoning. Each year, an estimated 33 to 50 million Americans get sick from foodborne bacteria, yeasts, molds, or viruses. The following steps will help keep your kitchen safe:

• Wash your hands before preparing food and after preparing raw meat or poultry; also wash your utensils, cutting board, and counter thoroughly with soap and hot water, especially after preparing raw meat or poultry.

• Use a fresh kitchen towel every time you cook.

• Keep pets away from food preparation areas.

• Marinate meats and poultry only in the refrigerator.

• Don't put cooked meat or poultry back into an uncooked marinade or serve the used marinade as a sauce unless you heat it to a rolling boil for several minutes.

• Hold foods at room temperature for no longer than an hour before or after cooking. Given the right conditions, the bacterial content in some foods can double in 20 minutes.

• Store starchy stuffing separately from the poultry in which it was cooked.

13 **Enrich your diet with beta carotene.** Beta carotene is the nutrient in fruits and vegetables that your body converts to vitamin A. Research suggests that beta carotene plays a role in preventing cancer. Rich sources include orange, yellow, and dark green fruits and vegetables such as carrots, sweet potatoes, mangos, cantaloupe, kale, watercress, and dandelion greens. Nutritionists recommend that your consume five to six milligrams of beta carotene a day; this requirement is easily met by eating a single carrot or half a cantaloupe.

14 **Dress your salad right.** Most commercial salad dressings, whether creamy or oily, get 90 percent of their calories from fat—

usually soybean oil. Some dressings also contain eggs, cream, and cheese. By making your own dressings at home, you can avoid much of the fat in commercial dressings:

- A creamy dressing can be made by mixing one and a half cups of plain nonfat yogurt, three tablespoons minced onion, three tablespoons chopped fresh dill, one minced garlic clove, one teaspoon dried oregano or basil, and pepper to taste.
- To cut fat and calories, use less oil and more vinegar when mixing a vinaigrette (the traditional ratio is three parts oil to one part vinegar). Try using flavorful walnut or dark sesame oil, and mild balsamic or rice vinegar, for a more palatable low-oil dressing. Add garlic, Dijon mustard, and herbs to vary the flavor.

15 **Select healthful snacks.** Pretzels contain practically no fat and, if you choose unsalted versions, very little sodium. Fig bars are among the best cookie choices around since they are low in fat and high in fiber. (They're high in sugar and calories as well, so don't eat more than a few at one sitting.) Graham crackers, too, are low in fat. Nuts are high in protein, vitamins, and minerals, but also in fat and calories; chestnuts, however, are the exception—one ounce of roasted chestnuts has just 69 calories and less than a gram of fat. Air-popped, unbuttered popcorn is one of the best snacks around; you would have to eat about 32 cups of it to get the 840 calories in a cup of peanuts. Another plus for popcorn: only about three percent of its calories come from fat, compared to 76 percent of the peanuts' calories. And popcorn is high in fiber. Try seasoning it with curry or onion powder (not onion salt), or other spices. Stay away from most store-bought bagged and microwave popcorns; most of these have added hydrogenated vegetable oil and may be just as high in fat as potato chips.

16 Choose foods rich in vitamin C. An adequate intake of vitamin C may help protect against cancer and possibly other diseases. The best way to get vitamin C is to eat fruits (or their juices) and vegetables such as asparagus, blackberries, broccoli, cantaloupe, cauliflower, cabbage, grapefruit, kale, kiwifruit, kohlrabi, mangoes, mustard greens, oranges, peppers, raspberries, strawberries, tangerines, and tomatoes.

17 Spice it up with healthy seasonings and condiments. Instead of using salt, substitute herbs (dill, oregano, basil, rosemary, thyme), spices (cumin, chili powder, curry powder, paprika), lemon or lime juice, or a combination of these. Mayonnaise contains very little cholesterol, but it is virtually 100 percent fat: try "light" or low-fat mayonnaise; or dilute mayonnaise with nonfat yogurt, lemon juice, or vinegar. Ketchup and mustard contain virtually no fat, but can be high in sodium—between 160 and 180 milligrams per tablespoon. Still, you can find low-sodium versions of both. Or you can substitute homemade salsa (a blend of chopped fresh tomatoes, chilies, onions, lime juice, and spices). Make your own mustard from dry mustard powder (you'll find basic directions on the package) and vary the flavor and texture by using milk or vinegar instead of water. Other low-fat, low-sodium condiment choices include horseradish, and apple, cranberry, or other fruit sauces. If you make fruit sauces at home, you can use much less sugar than store-bought products contain. Sweet pickle relish and chutney are good low-fat choices, but are often high in sodium.

18 Make whole-grain foods part of your diet. They're a nutritional bargain because whole grains are rich not only in vitamins and minerals but also fiber. In contrast, when wheat flour is refined, the fiber is removed and never replaced. Look for "100 percent whole wheat" on the label to make sure you are getting whole-grain bread. Buy brown rice and whole-grain cereals, too.

19 **Be a picky poultry eater.** By removing the skin from a chicken breast, you can cut its fat content by more than half. And choose the breast instead of the thigh: skinless dark meat contains more than twice as much fat as skinless light meat. It also has about 20 percent more calories and 10 percent less protein than light meat.

20 **Remember that vitamin E,** which plays an important role in maintaining healthy cells, may also help protect against cancer and other diseases. Plant oils (such as soybean, cottonseed, and sunflower) and products made from them (margarine, for example) are the richest sources; nuts, wheat germ, and green leafy vegetables are other good sources. Meats, fish, and fruits have small amounts. If your diet includes vegetable oils and green leafy vegetables, you'll undoubtedly get the recommended dietary allowance of vitamin E.

21 **Skim off fat.** There are many ways to defat foods:

- Use a bulb baster, a metal skimmer, or a long-handled spoon to skim the fat from gravies, sauces, and soups.
- Float a paper towel on top of hot soup to absorb fat, or blot it up with a wadded paper towel.
- Invest in a gravy separator. This inexpensive plastic device looks like a measuring cup with a spout attached in such a way that it drains the cup from the bottom. Pour in the pan juices, let them stand until the fat floats to the top, then pour off the defatted

juices through the spout and discard the fat that remains.

• Allow time to refrigerate sauces, soups, and gravies. As the liquid cools, the fat will rise to the top. When congealed, it can easily be removed. When using canned stock, sauce, or broth, refrigerate the can. When you take off the lid, the fat will be congealed on the surface and easy to remove.

22 **Eat fish to help your heart.** Eating even small amounts of fish (a serving or two a week) can significantly reduce the risk of heart attack. Scientists think that the protective value of fatty fish (such as salmon, sardines, and mackerel) is due to the type of polyunsaturated fatty acids, called omega-3s, found in its oil. The beneficial effect of omega-3s appears to come from their ability to reduce blood clotting.

23 **Pick low-fat sources of calcium.** An adequate calcium intake —especially during childhood and young adulthood—can help ward off osteoporosis, a disease characterized by a loss of bone mass that leaves bones brittle and more susceptible to fractures. Calcium requirements are as follows: ages 1 to 11—800 milligrams daily; ages 11 to 24—1,200 milligrams daily; and age 25 onward—800 milligrams per day. However, many experts believe that postmenopausal women—who are at greater risk for osteoporosis—should try to consume 1,200 to 1,500 milligrams of calcium per day. Dairy products are the best dietary sources of calcium, but whole-milk varieties, unfortunately, are also very high in fat. Choose low-fat or nonfat dairy products such as skim milk, low-fat or nonfat yogurt, and part-skim cheeses such as mozzarella and ricotta. These have as much calcium—and sometimes more—than their higher-fat counterparts. In addition, some vegetables (broccoli, Swiss chard, kale, mustard greens and spinach), canned salmon or sardines eaten with the bones, figs, almonds, soybeans, and tofu also provide good amounts of calcium. It's preferable not to depend on calcium supplements, however. Getting calcium through food ensures that you are also getting the other nutrients that work together to develop bone mass and help the body absorb calcium.

24 **Check out broccoli:** it's a powerhouse of nutrition. One cup of chopped cooked broccoli supplies 90 percent of the daily requirement of beta carotene, 200 percent of the vitamin C, significant amounts of niacin, calcium, thiamin, and phosphorus, and 25 percent of your fiber needs. Not only that, broccoli is one of the vegetables that may protect against certain forms of cancer. All this for only 45 calories.

25 **Eat a baked potato.** A large baked potato, eaten with the skin, contains only about 200 calories and is a good source of vitamin C (about half the daily requirement), B vitamins, iron, and potassium. It also contains some protein and a fair amount of fiber. Potatoes are unhealthful only when they are made into chips, hash browns, or fries, or topped with high-fat condiments like sour cream, butter, or cheese. Good low-fat toppings for potatoes include salsa and low-fat or nonfat plain yogurt.

26 **Eat more fiber.** Soluble fiber—found mostly in oats, legumes, fruits, and vegetables—helps lower blood cholesterol and manage blood sugar. Insoluble fiber is good for the digestive system and may protect against colon cancer; it is found primarily in wheat bran and whole grains. The recommended daily intake of dietary fiber from both types is 25 to 35 grams—equivalent to five servings of fruits and vegetables, and about six servings of breads, cereals, and legumes a day (servings are not large: one slice of bread, for instance, is considered a serving).

27 Know which fats you're eating. Saturated fat—abundant in beef, luncheon meats, whole-milk dairy products, butter, and tropical oils (coconut, palm, and palm kernel)—can elevate blood cholesterol levels and thus contribute to an increased risk of heart disease. The following is a sampling of unlikely places where saturated fats often lurk: packaged potato mixes, packaged rice dishes, stuffing/breading mixes, frozen vegetables in sauce, canned gravies, refried beans, crackers, bagel/pita bits, microwave popcorn, granola cereal, nondairy creamers, flavored instant coffee mixes, and toaster pastries. Polyunsaturated and monounsaturated fats—found in fish, nuts, and vegetable oils—do not have the same deleterious effect, and may actually lower cholesterol levels. This doesn't mean, however, that you should add these fats to your diet. Keep your total fat intake at or below 30 percent of your total daily calories; saturated fat should account for no more than a third of your total fat intake.

28 Boost your iron intake. Cooking in cast iron pots increases the iron content of foods. The more acidic the food (tomato sauce is highly acidic, for example), the more iron it will absorb. Another way to make the most of the iron you consume is to eat foods high in vitamin C at most meals. For instance, the vitamin C in your breakfast orange juice enhances your body's absorption of the iron in enriched cereal, and the presence of the vitamin in broccoli, tomatoes, leafy greens, and potatoes helps your body absorb the iron in the meats and legumes (such as beans, peas or lentils) you serve with these vegetables.

29 Eat beef wisely. Because of changes in the way cattle are bred, raised, and fed, beef is now significantly leaner than it was twenty years ago. But its fat content is widely variable. The best way to determine how much fat is in a piece of beef is to consider grade and cut. "Prime" is the fattiest, followed by "Choice" and "Select." "Select" meat has on average 20 percent less fat than "Choice," and 40 percent less fat than "Prime." Still, "Choice" beef can be low in fat, if you choose the right cuts. Top round, eye of round, London broil, and sirloin tip are the leanest. Whatever cut you choose, the best way to cut the fat content of beef is with a knife—trim all external fat before cooking.

Fitness

LEADING AN ACTIVE LIFE

30 Stretch before and after exercising, but don't stretch cold, tight muscles. Warm up first with five to six minutes of gentle exercise, such as jogging in place, stationary bicycling, or jumping jacks. When you've begun to perspire slightly or at least feel warm, it's safe to start stretching. Otherwise, you may cause microscopic tears in your muscles. Don't bounce when stretching, since this actually tightens muscles. The best kind of stretch is a "static" stretch, where you gradually increase the stretch without straining the muscles by holding the stretch for 10 to 15 seconds. Although recent studies have failed to show that stretching after a too strenuous workout heads off muscle soreness, it does promote flexibility and can keep your muscles from tightening up quickly.

31 **Work out in the water.** Swimming isn't the only kind of water exercise. Deep-water running and other water workouts can provide aerobic benefits without putting stress on joints and muscles. For people recovering from a leg or back injury, aquatic exercise is good because of the water's cushioning, supportive effect; this also makes it ideal for pregnant women or obese individuals. When exercising in water, make sure the temperature is comfortable, usually 82° to 86°. If it's too hot, you may feel weak or even pass out; if too cool, it may cause pain in stiff or arthritic joints.

32 **Mow your lawn aerobically.** Use an old-fashioned lawn mower rather than a power mower. Not only is it less expensive and less likely to break down, but it doesn't pollute the air. It also provides good exercise: pushing a manual mower for an hour burns between 420 and 480 calories—about as many as an hour of tennis.

33 **Know when to rest.** Many overuse injuries at first produce only mild or intermittent pain that you may be tempted to ignore, or that you may confuse with the twinges and mild muscle soreness that can accompany a strenuous workout (and that do not damage tissue). The telltale signs of a potentially serious injury include: severe or persistent muscle pain, swelling, or spasm; pain centered in a bone or joint; stiffness or decreased mobility of a joint; numbness or tingling. If any of these symptoms appear, you should stop exercising. Rest the affected muscles for at least five to seven days, then slowly return to training.

If the symptoms are severe or grow worse, consult your physician or a sports-medicine practitioner.

34 Take care of sore muscles. Stiff, sore muscles are common in weekend athletes who exercise only occasionally, as well as in frequent exercisers who suddenly increase the intensity of their workouts. This type of pain is called delayed-onset muscle soreness (DOMS). There is no proven treatment for DOMS, although recent research suggests that repeating the activity that caused the soreness—but at a much lower intensity—may ease discomfort. If DOMS becomes very uncomfortable and you want to take a pain reliever, don't reach for aspirin or ibuprofen, which may interfere with muscle repair and thus prolong soreness. These medications block the body's production of prostaglandins, substances that help stimulate the repair process. Acetaminophen (such as Tylenol), which has no anti-prostaglandin effect, is probably your best choice for the relief of muscle soreness. (However, aspirin or ibuprofen—such as Motrin or Advil—are the medications to take for the pain and inflammation of sprains, strains, and tendinitis.)

35 Underdress for winter workouts. The most common cold-weather problem for exercisers isn't that they wear too little clothing, but too much. Exercise raises body temperature significantly —even a moderate workout can make you feel like it's 30° warmer than it really is. So when you're about to run on a 25° day, dress for about 55°. It's a good idea to wear several layers that you can peel off as you become warm; clothes with zippers serve the same purpose. Wear a cap that you can stuff in your pocket when you're feeling comfortably warm.

36 **Buy the right athletic shoes.** Hold the front and back of the shoe and bend it. The sole should bend where the foot bends—at the ball; if it bends at mid-foot, it will offer little support. If your foot rolls outward significantly when you run, you're probably better off with a shoe that has a strong heel counter, a substantial yet somewhat soft mid-sole, a curved last, and a relatively flexible sole. If your foot tends to roll inward, you'll benefit from a shoe with a good arch support, a straight last, and a less flexible sole, especially along the inside.

37 **Eat to win.** The high-carbohydrate, low-fat diet that everyone should be eating for good health can actually help improve your athletic performance. Athletes who eat a diet that derives at least 70 percent of its calories from carbohydrates for the three days preceding a marathon race or other endurance event increase their muscles' ability to store glycogen—the muscles' storage form of the body's basic fuel, glucose. For a quick boost during an endurance event, a sugary pick-me-up like a candy bar or fruit drink may help replenish your energy stores. But remember, eating a sugary snack *before* the event is likely to be counterproductive; after a quick rise in blood sugar (and thus energy), your body responds by releasing insulin, which depresses your blood sugar level even lower than it was to start.

38 **Lift weights to become stronger.** Paired with regular aerobic exercise, weight training increases your strength and muscle endurance. Start weight training with light weights. If you belong to a gym, an exercise specialist there can help you develop a workout routine and teach you proper technique. Begin with a five to ten minute warm-up. At each session, do six exercises for the upper body and six for the lower body. Watch your breathing—exhale as your lift the weight, inhale as you lower it. Give each muscle group a full day of rest before exercising it again; exercising the same muscle group two days in a row may make it weaker, not stronger.

39 Walk, walk, walk. A study of thousands of Harvard alumni suggested that a long-term regimen of walking can significantly prolong life. Other research has shown that walking at speeds of three and a half to four and a half miles an hour—that's brisk walking, not strolling—produces cardiovascular benefits. Slower walking can be advantageous to older people, cardiac patients, or people recuperating from an illness. Walking at speeds of five miles an hour can burn as many calories as moderate jogging, but even slow walking can burn 60 to 80 calories per mile.

40 Get a stress test. An exercise stress test is an important diagnostic tool for uncovering cardiac problems. If the test indicates that you have a heart disorder, an appropriate exercise program can be designed for you. You should undergo a stress test before starting an exercise program if:

- You are 45 or over.
- You are between 35 and 44 and have at least one risk factor for coronary artery disease. (These include a parent or sibling who developed coronary artery disease before the age of 50, smoking, obesity, and elevated blood pressure or cholesterol level.)
- You have cardiovascular or lung disease at any age, or a metabolic disorder such as diabetes or hyperthyroidism. In these cases, the test itself may entail some risk, so you should consult your doctor first.

41 **Follow through on your exercise commitment.** Despite their best intentions, half of all people who take up new exercise programs drop by the wayside within six months. Here are some ways to bolster your perseverance:

• Set realistic, clear-cut exercise goals—say "I'll cycle ten miles this week" rather than "I really should get more exercise this week."

• Record your progress. Keep track of weight loss, exercise time, and heart rate.

• Start slow and easy. If you haven't exercised in some time, working out for ten minutes three times a week is easier than attempting four 45-minute sessions. Start at a moderate level, then gradually lengthen your workouts and step up the pace.

• Seek convenience. If the gym, track, or pool you use isn't nearby, you may use that as an excuse to stop exercising.

• Find a workout partner. One recent study found that 55 percent of women who exercised with a partner stuck with a twelve-month program versus only 31 percent of those who exercised alone.

• Add variety. Limiting yourself to one type of exercise day after day can become boring.

42 **Try cross-country skiing.** It's the best all-around aerobic sport there is. Using muscles in the shoulders, back, chest, abdomen, buttocks, and legs, cross-country skiers can burn 600 to 900 calories per hour. Champion cross-country skiers have set records for the highest levels of oxygen consumption ever, indicating excellent aerobic fitness. The kick-and-glide technique, combined with the poling motion to propel you along, can provide a more complete workout than running or cycling, which emphasize lower-body muscles. Cross-country skiing can also help develop coordination. And it has a lower risk of serious injury than downhill skiing.

43 **Pick the right sports drink.** Unless you are engaging in aerobic workouts lasting two hours or more, there is no evidence that sports drinks offer any advantage over water. Whatever drink you choose, it's important to replace lost fluids—even if you don't feel thirsty. In hot weather, drink at least 16 to 20 ounces of fluid two hours before exercising, and another 8 ounces 15 to 30 minutes before your workout. While you exercise, drink 3 to 7 ounces every 10 to 20 minutes. Drinks at 40° to 50° are absorbed more quickly than lukewarm beverages. After exercising, drink enough to replace the fluid you've sweated off: weigh yourself before and after your workout, and drink one pint for each pound lost.

44 **Take the stairs.** Make a point of climbing stairs instead of taking an elevator or escalator. As a supplement to other forms of exercise, stair climbing may help keep your weight in check while it strengthens your legs.

45 **Work all your major muscles.** Playing just one sport or performing just one type of exercise is likely to strengthen certain muscles at the expense of others, leaving some tendons and ligaments weaker and thus more vulnerable to injury. For example, shin splints—a common running injury that causes pain in the front of the lower leg—are often the result of an imbalance between the powerful muscles along the back of the lower leg and the relatively weaker ones in front. Varying your activities is one way to prevent this muscle imbalance. Another precaution is to conscientiously strengthen the muscle groups you underuse. And be sure to stretch all muscles involved in your workout.

46 Make sit-ups safe and effective. It's a myth that sit-ups—or any other abdominal exercise—can reduce observable fat around the waist, but they can strengthen and tone up your abdominal muscles, which are otherwise hard to exercise. Strong abdominal muscles may prevent or alleviate back problems, since they provide support for the back; they also provide additional power for running, tennis, and other physical exercises that involve the torso. Done improperly, however, sit-ups may actually strain the back and pelvis area, or work your leg and hip muscles more than your abdominal muscles. To do sit-ups safely and effectively, lie on the floor, keeping your knees bent and feet on the floor. Contract the abdominal muscles and press the lower back into the floor, which will cause the upper body to rise. It isn't necessary to lift your upper body beyond a 30° to 45° angle.

47 Cross train for health and pleasure. Alternating the types of sports or exercises you do may break the monotony of a one-exercise routine. Complementary workouts allow you to strengthen more muscle groups than a single activity would, and also allow each muscle group to rest while others get a workout. Some sports-medicine specialists also believe that cross training may reduce the risk of injury.

48 Wear a helmet when cycling. Head injuries account for 85 percent of the nation's 1,000 annual cycling deaths, 34 percent of which claim the lives of children aged 5 to 14. If everyone wore a helmet, many of the deaths would be prevented. Even if you're moving at only 20 miles an hour, if your unprotected head hits the pavement or a tree, you have little chance of surviving. Get a helmet approved by the American National Standards Institute (ANSI). A good one costs from $30 to $80.

49 Let yourself down easy with a push-up. The push-up remains one of the best upper-body exercises around. You can start with a modified version of the standard push-up called a "let-down." Begin in the up position of the standard push-up, with your arms fully extended and body straight. Bend your elbows and slowly lower yourself a few inches at a time, keeping your body aligned, until your chest is almost on the floor; this should take about 10 to 15 seconds. Kneel and relax for a moment, then return to the starting position and repeat. When the "let-down" becomes too easy for you, move on to the standard push-up.

50 Safeguard your knees. One out of every four sports injuries involves the knee. To prevent knee injuries, beware of suddenly intensifying your workouts, which can stress the knees and increase the risk of an overuse injury. Other factors that increase your chance of injury include worn-out or ill-fitting shoes and weak quadricep muscles (the muscles on the front of the thigh). Cycling is an excellent way to strengthen the quadriceps, as is walking up stairs or hills. If you're recovering from a knee injury, consult your doctor before undertaking any exercise.

51 Remember RICE for exercise injuries. For sprains, strains, and tendinitis: **R**est the injured part, apply **I**ce to the injured area for a maximum of 20 minutes, then re-apply it every two waking hours for the next 48 hours. Apply **C**ompression by wrapping a towel or an Ace-type bandage around the injury (but not so tightly that you cut off circulation). **E**levate the injured extremity above heart level.

52 **Put the right seat on your bicycle.** As you cycle, the whole of your weight rests on your two "sit bones," which in turn rest on the seat of your bike, so you may develop tenderness, chafing, bruising, or inflammation of the buttocks or crotch area. This is especially common among women, whose hip bones are usually about an inch wider apart than a man's so that standard bike seats are uncomfortable. Special anatomically designed saddles—wider and well cushioned at the back—can be helpful and are easy to install. Gel-filled or sheepskin saddles or pads can also ease the pressure and friction.

Stress Management

TAKING CARE OF YOUR MIND AND EMOTIONS

53 **Assess your job.** Studies have shown that workers who view themselves as simply "cogs in the wheel" experience more stress-related symptoms than those who see themselves as influential. In short, though "executive stress" exists, it's the bossed, not the bosses, who experience the most stress on the job. Work toward the goal of being an active participant at your job, rather than a passive observer. If you feel that your job does not allow you enough autonomy, make an attempt to change the situation. For a start, try to analyze what bothers you and come up with some possible solutions. Talk over your proposals with a co-worker. Next, speak to your supervisor. If you demonstrate skill at problem solving, your supervisor may show appreciation by giving you more responsibility. If, conversely, your job is managing others, you can reduce their stress by providing on-the-job training and offering real responsibilities that lead to a sense of control. If those who report to you seem bored and uninterested, remember that powerlessness can lead to stress and poor performance.

54 Boost your memory. Many people believe that memory loss is an unavoidable part of aging, but this doesn't have to be the case. You can keep your memory strong by keeping your mind active. Games—crossword puzzles, word games, and card games—are all good exercises for improving memory. Go to lectures, take night classes, or join activity groups; such pursuits will all introduce new stimuli. Develop tricks to improve your short-term memory: make up rhymes and compose mental pictures. Repeating and rehearsing new facts—such as the name of someone you've just met—can help, too.

55 Relax under pressure. Here are two simple relaxation techniques that can be done in a few minutes while you're at your desk, during your coffee break, or even while riding a bus.

- *Scanning.* Inhale and slowly "scan" your body, thinking about each muscle group (face and neck, shoulders, arms, abdomen, legs, and feet) and searching out tense muscles. As you exhale, relax the muscles that are tense.
- *Imagery.* Stop what you are doing and close your eyes. Imagine a beautiful scene. Spend a few minutes examining and enjoying every detail of the picture. See, hear, and smell pleasant things.

56 Don't drive yourself crazy while commuting. There are many ways to reduce the stress and strain of commuting. Try switching to public transportation or a car pool. If you must drive, see if you can adjust your work hours so that you don't have to travel at the height of the rush. Listen to educational tapes, audio books, or music to help you relax. And remember that responding angrily to other motorists only increases tension and makes your ride unpleasant. If your fellow motorist is clearly furious with you, check to see if you're doing something wrong. If so, try to correct it; if not, take a deep breath and ignore him.

57 Get a good night's sleep. If you frequently have trouble sleeping, try relaxing for an hour or so before getting into bed. Read, listen to music, take a warm bath (not a hot bath or forceful shower, which can be invigorating). Don't take work to bed with you. Avoid strenuous exercise within a couple of hours of bedtime. Cutting out caffeine-containing beverages and cigarettes before bedtime may also help; both are stimulants. Alcohol may help you fall asleep, but the sleep will probably be fragmented, light, and unsettled, and you're likely to wake up suddenly. Don't go to bed until you're sleepy, and if you can't fall asleep within 20 minutes or so, get out of bed and return only when you are sleepy. Repetitive, boring routines such as counting sheep may help you fall asleep. Or try to relax each muscle group, progressing slowly from your toes to your head. Get up at the same time every morning, no matter how poorly you've slept, and try to get through the day without a nap.

58 Write it out. Some research supports the belief that writing about problems or worries can be helpful. Other research has shown that holding back feelings about upsetting events can be psychologically harmful, and perhaps physically damaging as well. For people who have suffered experiences they are reluctant to discuss, or who have no ready listener, a session with pen and paper may serve as a comforting and useful substitute for talking.

59 Adjust your desk. A work area that is poorly fitted to your body can cause back, neck, and leg pain as well as fatigue. To alleviate discomfort, get a chair that can be adjusted to a height that allows your feet to rest comfortably on the floor (shorter people can put a footrest underneath the desk). The back of the chair should be 18 to 20 inches high to support your back. The desk should be 7 to 12 inches above the seat of the chair; the keyboard of your typewriter or computer should be 27 to 35 inches above the floor, approximately at elbow level when you're seated. While working, try to keep your shoulders relaxed and your head aligned with your spine. Leaning your head forward will put extra stress on the neck muscles.

60 Accentuate the positive. There is evidence that people who are hostile, cynical, or mistrustful are at increased risk for coronary artery blockages. Try to see the positive side of things and make time to pursue activities you enjoy. Researchers have found that one of the keys to reducing stress isn't just removing negative experiences from your life, but adding positive ones.

61 Reduce excess noise. According to government statistics, one out of every ten Americans in exposed to noise of sufficient intensity and duration to cause permanent hearing loss. There are many ways to reduce the noise in your environment. Play home and car stereos at reasonable levels. If you use headphones, don't turn the volume up so loud that it blocks external sounds. Hang overlapping, double drapes over the windows to block outside noise; upholstered furniture will help absorb sound indoors. If the kitchen is noisy, install sound-absorbing ceiling tiles, and place rubber pads under noisy appliances such as blenders. Wear earplugs when operating loud equipment such as drills or chainsaws, and when attending highly amplified music performances. You can also wear earplugs if street noise is intolerable.

Safe Travel

HEALTH AND SAFETY AWAY FROM HOME

62 Know your hotel. There are, on average, 8,000 hotel fires in the U.S. each year, in which dozens of people die, most of them from inhaling smoke and toxic fumes, not from burns. It's wise to know the location of your floor's fire alarm, and at least two possible escape routes from your floor. Count the number of doors between your room and the nearest exit. In the event of a fire, this will allow you to feel your way there through darkness or smoke.

63 Ease jet lag. Jet lag is caused by a disruption of sleep/wake patterns. Flying westward lengthens your day, and flying eastward shortens it. Because it compresses the day/night cycle, the eastward flight is more likely to produce jet lag. One preventive technique is to start shifting your sleep/wake cycle to the new time in advance. If traveling east to west, go to bed—and get up—an hour later each day for three days before departure. For a west-to-east trip, move your sleep time an hour earlier each day. If traveling great distances, schedule a stopover if you can. Once you arrive, sunlight may help reset your biological clock. Spend some time outdoors during the first few days. And despite tiredness or wakefulness, try to go to sleep and get up at your usual hours.

64 **Steer clear of ice cubes in countries where the water is unsafe.** Treat ice cubes in developing countries with just as much caution as you would the drinking water. When contaminated ice cubes are allowed to melt in beverages—alcoholic or otherwise—enough bacteria can survive to cause traveler's diarrhea. If you're making your own ice cubes and safe water is unavailable, boil tap water for two to three minutes.

65 **Fly comfortably.** The cabin air of an airplane is thinner and dryer than normal air, so it's best to avoid alcohol, which dehydrates you. Drink lots of non-alcoholic liquids, even if you're not thirsty. And get up to stretch and walk around once an hour, since sitting for long periods can hamper digestion, circulation, and flexibility, and can also cause your feet to swell.

66 **Buy a car with an airbag.** If all Americans used lap-and-shoulder belts *and* all cars were equipped with airbags, an estimated 9,000 lives would be saved annually, and 150,000 serious injures prevented. If you're shopping for a car, let the car dealer know you're interested in an airbag. Even though airbags don't come with every car, you can exert your influence for change. Even if your car has an airbag, remember to wear your safety belt, too.

67 Maintain healthy eating habits when you travel. One survey showed that frequent business travelers tend to eat a diet higher in fat (45 to 48 percent of their total calories coming from fat) than other groups. And no wonder: travelers often have few options (on planes, for example, or at fast-food outlets) or may find gourmet restaurant fare irresistible. But there are ways to control your eating habits away from home. For example, airlines are required to offer special meals, provided passengers place their orders 24 hours in advance. You can often get low-calorie, low-cholesterol, low-sodium, vegetarian, diabetic, or kosher meals—just ask what's available. Or if you prefer, pack your own low-fat meal. In restaurants, good starters include a broth-based soup, steamed seafood, fresh melon, or a green salad (have the dressing served on the side). Choose foods that are poached, steamed, broiled, or roasted, and ask that butter or oil be used sparingly (or not at all) in the cooking. Ask to have the skin removed from poultry before cooking, or remove it yourself when the dish arrives. Sauces such as hollandaise, mayonnaise, tartar sauce, and rémoulade are all high in fat. Brown sauces, such as bordelaise or bourguignonne, are stock-based and may be lower in fat if they have been skimmed and no butter has been added. Meatless tomato sauces are likely to be relatively low in fat.

68 Wear your seat belt. Seat belts saved nearly 11,000 lives in the U.S. between 1983 and 1987, according to federal officials. By wearing a lap-and-shoulder belt, you reduce your risk of dying in an automobile accident by 40 to 50 percent.

69 Choose a car with antilock brakes. Antilock brakes may one day contribute substantially to highway safety. Activated by a sensor attached to each car wheel, these brakes detect potential skids and react accordingly, pulsing the brake power and bringing the vehicle to a faster, safer stop than conventional brakes. Antilock brakes are now standard equipment on some cars and optional on some others.

Self Care

ADDRESSING COMMON HEALTH CONCERNS

70 Rehydrate your skin. Dry skin is a common problem, particularly in the winter, when cold dry air, wind, and dry indoor heat can parch your skin. Skin also becomes drier with age. Simple moisturizers (free of perfumes, colors, thickeners, or emulsifiers, which can cause sensitivity reactions) may help; they form a thin film of oil that holds moisture to your skin, thus protecting you from drying conditions. In addition, you can add a little bath oil to your bath water. Bathe or shower in tepid water and use a mild soap to avoid washing away the natural oils that help trap water in your skin. Apply a light coating of moisturizer immediately after bathing to take advantage of your skin's dampness. In cold weather, wear gloves and cover your face with a scarf or ski mask.

71 Stay out of tanning salons. Any tan caused by ultraviolet light—whether from the sun or a sun lamp—damages the skin and greatly increases your risk of developing skin cancer later in life. Tanning salons are unregulated in most states and are as unsafe as ever. The greatest danger of a sunlamp may be to the eyes. If used without protective goggles, sun lamps can burn the sensitive skin of your eyelids, or cause temporary or even permanent blindness. Keeping your eyes closed is not sufficient protection.

72 Prevent nighttime calf cramps. If you seem predisposed to nocturnal calf cramps, don't point your toes while stretching in bed, and try not to sleep with your toes pointed. Sleep on your side, since people who lie on their back or stomach tend to keep their toes pointed. Don't tuck in your blankets and sheets too tightly—they can bend your toes down. When a cramp occurs, your best bet for relief is stretching and massage. Simply stretch your foot (and, by extension, your calf muscles) by flexing your toes upwards. Grasping your toes and the ball of your foot and pulling them up may help. At the same time, massage the calf muscles gently. Walking may help, too, particularly if you put your full weight on your heels. Ice packs can reduce blood flow and thus relax muscles. A helpful stretch: stand two to three feet from a wall and face it; lean your weight on your forearms against the wall for 15 to 20 seconds, keeping your heels on the floor.

73 Keep lead out of your water. Nearly one in five Americans, in all parts of the country, drinks water with lead levels considered excessive by the Environmental Protection Agency. Homes built more than 80 years ago may still contain pipes made of lead or lead alloy. If your pipes contain lead, you can reduce the amount of lead in your tap water by letting the water run for a few minutes in the morning to flush out standing water that has been in contact with any lead plumbing materials. Don't drink, cook, or prepare baby formulas with hot tap water, since hot water dissolves lead more quickly than cold. And if you have any new plumbing installed, insist that nonlead materials be used.

74 Take steps to prevent colds. The most effective way to avoid catching a cold (or spreading one) is hand washing. Wash your hands often and avoid putting your fingers to your nose and eyes. Try not to share objects—such as telephones, cups, or pencils—with cold sufferers. And don't rely on vitamin C; no study has ever shown it to be an effective cold preventive, and megadoses can lead to nausea, abdominal cramps, and diarrhea.

75 Microwave safely. Microwave ovens tend to preserve vitamins better than conventional cooking methods because they cook foods so quickly. But this type of cooking may heat foods unevenly and leave some parts undercooked, allowing bacteria and other microorganisms to survive. To avoid this problem:

• Cover cooking vessels with glass or ceramic lids (or plastic wrap made to be used in microwave ovens); the trapped steam will cook the surface of the food while the microwaves are cooking the inside. Be sure to leave the lid slightly ajar, or prick a hole in the plastic wrap to vent the steam.

• Allow microwaved food to stand after the cooking time is over. Heat concentrated inside the food will radiate outward, cooking the exterior and equalizing the temperature. Food will taste better this way, too, since it will be consistently hot throughout.

• Thaw meats before cooking them (most microwaves can also defrost foods). Ice crystals are not heated well by microwaves and can leave cold spots.

76 Avoid unnecessary dental X-rays. Oral X-rays shouldn't be a routine procedure, but instead ordered only to diagnose specific conditions. Whenever you do get dental X-rays, always request a lead apron and collar for optimal protection.

77 Remember that adults need immunizations. You need a *tetanus* booster every 10 years. (If you sustain a heavily contaminated wound, see a doctor: a booster may be appropriate if you have not received one within the preceding five years.) Anyone over 65 is advised to get an *influenza* vaccination yearly since strains of influenza vary from year to year. Anyone with chronic pulmonary, heart, or kidney disease or diabetes should also be vaccinated for influenza. These same groups should also receive a one-time vaccine against the 23 strains of bacteria that cause about 80 percent of the pneumococcal diseases (predominantly pneumonia) in this country. People born after 1957, who were vaccinated between 1963 and 1967, may have gotten a short-lasting *measles* vaccine and should be revaccinated. Women of child-bearing age who have no history of a *rubella* (German measles) vaccination should be tested for antibodies and, in their absence, be immunized. A woman should wait at least three months after this vaccination before becoming pregnant.

78 Block UV light with sunglasses. Up to 100,000 of the million cataract cases reported each year in the U.S. may be sun-related and thus preventable. Surprisingly, you can protect your eyes from the sun's damaging ultraviolet (UV) rays with a pair of sunglasses that cost less than $10. It's not true that dark sunglasses cause your pupils to dilate and thus admit more UV rays. Gray and green lenses are the least likely to distort colors (traffic lights, for example); amber and brown are also acceptable. Other lens colors, such as red, blue, and purple, tend to distort colors too much. Look for sunglasses that carry American National Standards Institute (ANSI) labels, and look for models that block at least 95 percent of UV rays.

79 Prevent heartburn. Don't overeat. Avoid tight clothing, especially waist-pinching belts. Stay upright for several hours after eating—don't eat just before bedtime or lie down for a nap right after a meal. If you frequently suffer from heartburn, avoid chocolate, alcohol, tomatoes, and citrus fruits. Limit fat intake, since fat slows the emptying of the stomach. Elevate the head of your bed by six inches or more (use wood blocks or thick telephone books); this may be the single most important mechanical alteration heartburn sufferers can make.

80 Keep your garden pesticide-free. Most gardeners are now aware that chemical pesticides can endanger human health as well as kill insects. There are more cons than pros to using pesticides in home gardens, and if you keep your garden healthy, you won't need them. Choose a garden site in a well-drained area, and don't overwater. Pull weeds regularly. Plant marigolds, nasturtiums, garlic, onions, or chives around the garden border; they help repel some insects. Buy insect- and disease-resistant seedlings when possible.

81 Give your teeth five minutes each day. Carefully brush your teeth at least twice a day and use dental floss. Regularity and thoroughness of brushing are the keys to removing plaque. Flossing is just as important as brushing for healthy teeth and gums. Dental floss is available in different thicknesses and flavors, which may help make flossing your teeth a more regular habit.

82 Get a Pap smear. Pap smears can detect cervical cancer at the earliest possible stage, and when caught early, cervical cancer is nearly 100 percent curable. A woman should have her first Pap smear at age 18 or when she becomes sexually active. According to the U.S. Preventive Services Task Force, if her test results are normal for three consecutive years, she can undergo less frequent screenings, generally every three years, at the discretion of her doctor. However, women at high risk for cervical cancer—those who smoke, have genital warts or other sexually transmitted diseases, or have frequent sex with many partners—should have annual Pap smears.

83 **Give yourself a testicular exam.** Testicular cancer is the leading form of cancer in young men between 29 and 35—although it's rare, comprising only one percent of all cancers. Fortunately, the survival rate approaches 100 percent if the cancer is detected early enough. Men should give themselves a monthly testicular exam. After a warm shower or bath, when the scrotal skin is relaxed, gently roll each testicle between the thumb and fingers of both hands to feel for lumps, nodules, swelling, or a change in consistency in the testicles. Abnormalities warrant a doctor's attention.

84 **Get a mammogram.** A mammogram—an X-ray of the breast—is one of the most valuable tools for the early detection of breast cancer. Women between ages 35 and 40 should get a "baseline" mammogram for later comparison. Women between the ages of 40 and 49 should have a breast X-ray every year or two, and have annual mammograms after age 50.

85 **Wear a sunscreen.** There has been an "epidemic" increase (more than 300 percent) in the incidence of the two deadly forms of skin cancer—malignant melanoma and squamous cell skin cancer—since 1960. The best way to reduce your risk of developing skin cancer is to wear a waterproof sunscreen with a sun protection factor (SPF) of 15 or more every time you go out in the sun. Look for a "broad-spectrum" sunscreen, which contains two or more ingredients that absorb ultraviolet light. And make sure your kids (over the age of six months) are equally well protected. Skin damage from the sun is cumulative, and according to one estimate, most Americans have received 78 percent of their lifetime exposure to the sun by the age of 20.

86 **Wipe out allergens.** Nearly 30 million Americans suffer from hay fever, according to the National Center for Health Statistics. If you suffer from allergies, remember that allergens are most prevalent between 5 a.m. and 10 a.m. Use an air conditioner, if your have one, but keep its filter clean, or you may end up blowing allergens around the house. (For your car's A/C, try keeping your car windows partially open for 10 to 15 minutes after you turn it on. If this doesn't help, have your car treated with the EPA-registered disinfectant called RenNew-A/C, available at car-dealer service departments, some service stations, and most auto A/C shops.) Keep your house cool, but not cold, since too-cold temperatures may aggravate your runny nose and other allergy symptoms. Avoid alcohol and tobacco smoke, which can also aggravate allergic conditions.

87 **Watch your back.** About 80 percent of all Americans will have at least one backache during their lifetime. Backaches can arise from a variety of causes: excess body weight, poor posture, standing or sitting in one position for long periods, sleeping on your stomach (which makes the stomach sag and increases swayback), lifting and carrying heavy objects, wearing girdles or tight pants (which promote weak abdominal muscles), or wearing high heels (which tend to increase the curvature of the back). Psychological stress may also contribute to muscle tension in the lower back and elsewhere, and tense muscles are more susceptible to injury.

88 **Know your cholesterol level.** If you haven't been tested, ask your doctor or call your local hospital, health department, or the local chapter of the American Heart Association for advice about when and where to get a test. Don't get a "finger-stick" test at the local mall or supermarket, where conditions are often unsanitary and results unreliable.

89 **Choose shoes that fit.** Ill-fitting shoes are thought to cause 80 percent of all foot problems. To find a comfortable pair, shop for shoes in the middle of the day, not early in the morning, since your feet swell as the day progresses. Wear the kind of socks or stockings that you intend to wear with the shoes. To ensure proper fit, ask to have both feet measured (the metal Brannock device is more accurate than a wooden ruler), and always put your full weight on the foot being measured. Try the size that fits the larger foot. Remember, sizes indicate very little: size 8½ C in one brand may be a 9 B in another. Imported shoes are likely to run small. You should never buy a shoe with the idea of breaking it in. The shoe may alter your foot (for instance, causing corns, calluses, and blisters), rather than the reverse.

90 **Keep an eye on your birthday suit.** Check your skin monthly for any signs of skin cancer. To distinguish a normal mole from an abnormal one, use the ABCD rule: Asymmetry—one half of the mole doesn't match the other; Border—it is irregular, or has ragged or bumpy edges; Color—the mole is several colors or has changed color; and Diameter—the mole is growing in size, or is larger than about six millimeters across (the size of a pencil eraser). Also see a doctor if you have: a sore that doesn't heal in three weeks; a persistent reddish patch; a smooth bump indented in the middle with rolled borders; or a shiny, waxy, scarlike spot without regular borders.

91 **Protect your voice.** Your vocal cords react just like any other tissue strained by overuse: they resist. If you do get hoarse, speak only when absolutely necessary and in a soft, breathy voice. Don't whisper—it puts more tension on your vocal cords than speaking softly. To prevent hoarseness:

• Avoid talking over background noise.

• Speak softly when using the telephone. If you have to be on the phone for long periods, a phone rest or headset may lessen the strain on muscles in your face, throat, and neck, thus reducing tension on your vocal cords.

• Don't pitch your voice unnaturally high or low.

• Keep your vocal cords well lubricated by increasing your fluid intake and the humidity of indoor air.

92 **Check your night vision.** Few people realize that even though they may have 20/20 vision in the daytime, their nighttime vision will have deteriorated considerably by the time they turn 40. Try to reduce the number of nighttime driving trips you make. If you must drive at night, drive more slowly and carefully. Unless there is another car approaching, use your high beams (but remember that your headlights may temporarily blind a pedestrain.) Keep your dashboard lights low so that your eyes are not constantly readjusting from light to darkness.

93 Use a humidifier in the winter. Indoor heat dries out the air, and dry air in turn reabsorbs moisture from any available source —your skin, your throat, and the interior of your nose, as well as your furniture and houseplants. A dry throat and nose are uncomfortable in themselves, can make a cold more annoying, and can irritate the lungs. Moreover, dry mucous membranes may make you more susceptible to colds. The best way to combat this is to use an ultrasonic humidifier. Unlike cool-air humidifiers, they eject no live molds and very few bacteria into the air. If possible, use distilled water in your ultrasonic humidifier. If you use tap water, run it through a demineralizing filter first, since tap water contains minerals that can be dispersed into the air by the humidifier and then inhaled into the deepest part of the lungs. This can actually increase your susceptibility to colds and flu as well as aggravating chronic respiratory diseases like asthma and bronchitis.

94 Fire-proof your hearth. Take steps to cut down on creosote, a tarlike substance that may accumulate in a chimney and catch fire there, possibly cracking the chimney or setting fire to the house. If you use your fireplace often, have the chimney inspected annually and, if necessary, cleaned. Build small, hot fires rather that large smoky ones to reduce creosote buildup. Use well-seasoned wood (stored and dried for at least six months). Hardwood (such as maple, oak, or elm) is preferable because it produces a steady, long-lasting blaze. You may want to use some softwood (pine, spruce, or fir) as a starter, since it is easier to ignite, but don't use too much: it burns faster and sparks more, increasing the risk of a chimney fire. Don't burn colored papers or plastic, which can produce harmful fumes. Artificial logs contain wax and coloring agents and thus make a dirtier fire, contributing to creosote buildup; if you use them, burn only one at a time, and place it on a grate.

95 Seek social support. Social interactions with family, friends, the community, and co-workers can be a factor in maintaining health. Studies have shown that people who enjoy the companionship of friends and family live longer and are healthier than people who are socially isolated.

96 Chew sugarless gum when you can't brush. Gum-chewing stimulates copious secretions of saliva, and saliva helps neutralize tooth-decaying acids in dental plaque. The chewing action also helps pump saliva into the spaces between teeth. For maximum effect, chew a piece of sugarless gum within 15 minutes of finishing a meal and chew for 15 to 20 minutes. Any more than that can cause jaw pain, erode biting surfaces, crack fillings, and loosen dental inlays.

97 Protect yourself from sexually transmitted diseases. Use latex condoms and a spermicide containing nonoxynol-9 (these do not provide infallible protection, but do weigh the odds significantly in your favor). Be observant: don't have sexual contact with anyone who has genital or anal sores, a visible rash, a discharge, or any other sign of venereal disease. Be selective and know your partner; it's risky to have sexual intercourse with someone you've just met. Be informed: if you think you've been exposed to a sexually transmitted disease (STD), don't have sex again until you've seen a doctor and been diagnosed and, if necessary, treated. Remember that syphilis, like AIDS, can be transmitted by contaminated needles used in tattooing, acupuncture, even ear piercing. Make sure such instruments are sterile (or disposable). Inform your children about STDs: sex education in school can help, but there's no substitute for parent-child discussions about sexuality.

98 Take a break from your computer. Working at a computer for hours on end can cause eyestrain, and neck and back strain. To prevent these symptoms, get up every 40 minutes or so and stretch, walk around, or do simple relaxation exercises. You'll be able to work more efficiently if you are relaxed and comfortable.

99 Join a support group to stop smoking. Some would-be quitters may find comfort in knowing that there are others out there wrestling with the same problem. The support of a group may give you the impetus you need to finally kick the habit. Free or inexpensive quit-smoking support groups, sponsored by the American Lung Association and the American Cancer Society, are available in many areas. Check your telephone directory for the local chapter.

100 Protect the ozone layer to protect yourself. The Environmental Protection Agency estimates that for every one-percent decrease in the ozone layer in the stratosphere, the incidence of skin cancers will increase between three and six percent. The ozone layer is being destroyed in large part by manmade compounds called chlorofluorocarbons (CFCs). The following steps can help reduce CFC emissions:

• Have your car's air conditioner carefully serviced. Auto air conditioners are the single largest source of CFC emissions in the U.S. Don't simply refill your leaky air conditioner; if you don't have the leak fixed, the CFCs you add will end up in the air. Go to a service station equipped to recycle CFCs.

• Don't use foam plastic insulation in your home, unless it is made with ozone-safe agents.

• Don't buy a halon fire extinguisher for home use.

• When buying a refrigerator, choose an energy-efficient model: it may contain as little as half as much CFCs as other models.

101 **Install smoke detectors.** Smoke detectors significantly reduce your chances of being injured or killed in a fire. Put a smoke detector in every room of your house (except the bathroom), the basement and attic included. Detectors should be mounted high on a wall or on the ceiling, but at least four inches from where the wall and ceiling meet. Don't mount smoke detectors within three feet of a window, door, or vent, since drafts and water vapor can prevent smoke from reaching the device. There are three types of detectors: ionization devices—the most common type—which are most sensitive to fast-burning fires and react quickly to cooking smoke; photoelectric devices, which are more expensive but react faster to the kind of smoldering fire that begins, for example, in wiring or upholstery, and less quickly to cooking smoke; and combination units, which respond to all kinds of fires, and are thus the best choice if you're choosing only one unit. You can put a photoelectric device in the kitchen (it's less likely to "cry wolf" every time you burn toast), and combination or ionization detectors in most other areas of your home.

The *University of California, Berkeley Wellness Letter* is published monthly by Health Letter Associates: *Rodney M. Friedman,* Editor and Publisher; *Shirley Abbott Tomkievicz,* Editorial Director; *Michael Goldman,* Executive Editor; *Dale A. Ogar,* Managing Editor; *Bette Ponack Albert, M.D.,* Medical Editor; *Jeanine Barone, M.S.,* Sports Medicine and Nutrition Editor; *Jane Margaretten-Ohring, R.N.,* Associate Medical Editor; *Barbara Maxwell O'Neill,* Associate Publisher; *Karin Anderson,* Assistant Editor.

Staff for this book: *Karin Anderson,* Executive Editor; *Patricia Calvo,* Senior Editor; *Bonnie J. Slotnick,* Copy Editor; *Andrea Ross,* Designer.